DIABETES:

The Ultimate Step-By-Step Guide to Reverse Diabetes Forever and Have Long-Lasting Success

by

Hannah Parkes

Table of Contents

Chapter 7-conclusion

Chapter 1-Introduction

This is a topic that has been covered over and over again and the purpose of this book is not to re-hash what has already been said in the same way. I will attempt during the course of this book to provide a different view of "diabetes" and more specifically what it means to someone who has diabetes. This also applies to someone who is pre-disposed to developing diabetes either through their existing lifestyle choices or otherwise. I use the term "condition" instead of "disease" for a very good reason. It is all about context, and how we choose to see things.

In todays modern world everything is labeled, debated and just about everything has some sort of "spin" on it to borrow a marketing term. So we hear about the horror stories, the fact that it is a "silent killer", it is on the rise and it is going to wipe out half the population! Is it actually going to wipe out half the population? According to UK statistics from the NHS (National Health Service) 3.9 million people live with it in the UK. It is projected that around 5 million people will be in this position by 2025 in the UK alone. Let's just unpack this for a moment. The UK currently has 65 million people living in it. So with 3.9 million diabetes sufferers this would mean in the region of 6% of the population. If we assume the same average for the world population it would mean that about 446 million people worldwide suffer from diabetes as a rough estimate. The question of if this is a problem that needs to be addressed is self-explanatory. But is this problem some disease that's arrived in the modern world to kill us and exact a heavy price? I do not believe so in the least.

This is a "condition" that more and more people are suffering from and is not a "silent killer" as sometimes described, but rather something that is a symptom / result of an unbalanced and unhealthy lifestyle. Being only defined as the specific condition "diabetes" in the early 1900's when its root cause was discovered, it has been around for a long time dating back to Egyptian times when its symptoms were first recorded. The point is not its existence but more about how wide spread it has become. Now is when the "context" that was mentioned earlier starts to become apparent. The "context" is our lives, our lifestyles, what we eat, how we eat, what we do and how and when we do it. These are the things that have changed.

This leads to the conclusion that it's about our environment, and how we live in that environment that is helping diabetes become more prevalent. If that is the case, then surely by paying attention to all of these things, we can adjust, correct and change aspects of our lives to have the reverse effect. By this I mean, take out all the things that are making it easier to suffer from diabetes and replace them with all the things that make it difficult for this condition to even manifest let alone continue unabated. It is from these conclusions, that the idea of diabetes being reversed originates. However, as you will see in later chapters, there is a form of diabetes that cannot be tackled purely this way, which is Type-1 diabetes.

Today's Food:

We have all seen and heard of the "fads" in today's modern world regarding food. As an example, look at a recipe book from the 70's for healthy eating, and then look at a recipe book from the modern day on the same topic. Some things may look familiar, but the general feeling and overall picture is very different. This highlights that over the years its not so much our ability to judge what is good or not good food, but rather it is a very good example of how much better food production companies have become at convincing us that what they are selling us is better and healthier.

The opposite is actually true! The food we are consuming is getting worse and worse as far as quality and health benefits. It is a "profit" driven business model that is not so much concerned with health benefits but rather the profit margin. Unfortunately some of the casualties of this change in modern culture are the people who now suffer from diabetes. As an example we consume more sugar through variety of foods than we have ever done before, in some cases as much as 60kg of refined sugar per person per year! At least half of the sugar we consume we don't even know we are taking in. It is found in bread, processed meat products and fruit juices are a particularly nasty example of this massive use of refined sugar. We have been conditioned into believing that fruit and therefore fruit juice is healthy. In some cases, one small carton of fruit juice contains the entire recommended daily allowance of sugar for a full grown adult. That's it, just one small carton of fruit juice and that's it, no more sugar for the day!

We consume more synthetically made food products than ever before. "Processed" has become a dirty word and for very good reasons. "Refined" is another prime example, it's supposed to mean "better food" but it is for all intents and purposes another very good marketing strategy that has been used over the years to sell cheaper and generally less healthy food. Even actively looking for healthier food products in today's modern supermarket, does not mean it is anywhere near as healthy for our bodies as say similar products 20 or 30 years ago. Too many products on the shelf, in restaurants and generally available for us to eat, have in some way been processed and refined. This invariably means they have lost some or all of the "healthy" components that we think we are actually buying. This also means they contain substantially more of the unhealthy things that we should be avoiding.

So is "eating the right way" going to be the answer? Unfortunately not on its own, because even when you are actively trying by choosing your diet carefully, the prevalence of processed and refined food products means we don't have the quality and variety that we used to be able to choose from. It is harder to eat better, and in some countries especially so. My personal experience has shown me that even eating correctly, I had to do something more to maintain a healthy balance. Fresh is better, organic is even better. Processed or refined lead to unbalanced diets and the problems caused by them.

Today's Lifestyle:

This next chapter delves into another very powerful driver of "conditions" such as diabetes. Lifestyle! By using the word lifestyle I am broadening the scope to include not just exercise, but how we live on a day to day basis in modern first world life and how this evolution of lifestyle has some unfortunate downsides. Firstly, the modern working week averages between 30 to 50 hours per week. Traveling to and from work is becoming harder and longer as population centers grow and become more congested. This adds more time. We have our social lives, and the growing consumption of digital media, which again takes time, just to name a few. By looking at time as a finite resource, an average persons week is becoming more and more crowded, busier and busier and generally people seem to have less and less time. A result of this is that less and less time is given to what we eat, how we prepare it and where we get it. Fast food has come of age in the modern day purely because people have less time to grow their own vegetables, wash and prepare their own food, go to 10 different shops in the local area for fresh produce. The reason is because it's easier and "faster" to get it all in one place, that takes as little time to get done as possible. It seems like a win-win but is it? Yes its easier and faster, but the cost can be life changing, especially if you find out that well, you have now got Type-2 diabetes.

Physical activity is one of the most important aspects. This does not just mean exercise and getting your daily dose of cardio. It is your entire 24-hour cycle of activity. If you spend 35 hours a week sitting behind a desk, it follows that you would need to do substantially more physical activity than say a tour guide who walks people around a national park every day. We need to be consciously aware of what kind of daily life we have and how we find a balance that includes a quality amount of physical activity. The human body is designed to move, if it was designed to sit in a chair I believe we would look very different than we do today. A lack of regular physical activity and movement means our body slows down, the biological machine that is our body starts going into what I would call a stasis mode. These changes the body's chemistry, which in turn means it becomes unbalanced if this occurs for excessive or prolonged periods of time. As well as the lack of time we have for paying attention to what we eat we seem to have less time to be physically active. A picture is beginning to build showing how lopsided a modern day life can actually become.

Today's Stress:

Stress is natural. It's not just some modern day symptom of an intense and busy lifestyle. Stress and more specifically, the way our bodies react to stress is a biological mechanism that is a part of us. The effect on our body is immediate when we are in a stressful situation and the following happens. Our bodies release hormones in response to stress. This elevates our heart rate and breathing giving our bodies more oxygen. This is like a "turbo-boost" to use a simple analogy. Our brains function faster, our muscles react with increased power to name a few immediate benefits. The problem arises when we experience stress constantly. In modern day terms this is defined as chronic stress. To compound this problem, most people don't even realize they have constant stress levels. Modern lifestyles inherently generate constant pressure, which turns into constant stress. Chronic stress is a widely recognized driver in many modern day conditions including irregular and unhealthy eating patterns. Stress has a part to play in pre-disposing people who are susceptible to developing diabetes.

What this means:

What this means is that it's not just someone's body that does not perform properly. It is not just a lack of exercise on a regular basis such as going to the gym three times a week for an hour. It is not just eating healthy organic food prepared lovingly at home with only the best natural produce money can buy. It is not just living a stress free life without a care in the world. There is no one-fix solution as there is no one-source problem. It is the combination of all these things and more that create a pre-disposition to becoming diabetic. It follows that by addressing all of these factors together in a combined way, yes absolutely it is possible to prevent diabetes from taking hold and if you already have the condition, it is possible to manage it and keep it stable and also to go as far as eventually eradicating the condition all together. It is about our bodies, which as amazing and complex and wonderful as they are, need to be looked after.

Chapter 2-How does it work?

Our Body – biological wonder machine:

Our bodies are wonderful, complex and beautiful works of evolutionary art. They can perform incredible feats of physical prowess and mental dexterity. We have conquered every corner of our planet, not just with our minds but because we have the physical abilities and bodies to do so. In order for such an incredible biological machine to work, its complexity has to be just as incredible. Without diving into the full scope of human anatomy, the focus will be on a particular aspect. What we call processes and systems. The human body has a host of control systems or processes that control a whole variety of things, from how we obtain and use oxygen to how we feel. The main systems are things such as the endocrine system, digestive system and the nervous system.

The endocrine system is the key player that will be discussed here and is affectionately known as the "hormonal system". This system communicates with the rest of the body by using a form of chemical messaging (hormones) much like the nervous system uses neural (electrical) messaging. These messages generally trigger an increase or decrease of activity in the part of the body being targeted. The point of this control system is to maintain homeostasis or what I will refer to as a "balanced state". For a diabetic the core of the problem lies in how one of these systems works or should we say stops working properly. The organ responsible is the pancreas, the two hormones involved are insulin and glucagon and it's all about how the blood sugar (glucose) levels are controlled.

Control Systems – active chemical control systems:

A very basic explanation of the how these components work together is as follows. When we exercise, our muscles need fuel, which happens to be a form of sugar called glucose. As our muscles use this glucose, the levels of glucose in our blood drop. Our Pancreas responds when it detects the lower glucose levels by secreting a short burst of glucagon (stimulator in this case). This causes the liver to release more glucose into the blood. The body gets back to its normal state or as we say it re-attains homeostasis. The opposite action is when the glucose levels are too high, for example when we have a sugar spike, but don't need all the glucose floating around in our blood stream. Again our pancreas reacts but this time it secretes a burst of insulin (inhibitor in this case). This causes fat cells in the body to start storing the glucose, and so again, the body takes itself back to a balanced state. This is how the system works normally.

What happens when it goes wrong and why does it go wrong!!

So why does this system go wrong? This question has a two-part answer, as there are two types of diabetes and both for slightly different reasons. Of the two main types of diabetes the most common one is Type-2 diabetes. The cause of which is generally understood. Type-1 diabetes is a different thing altogether as no proven cause has yet been agreed on. In the pancreas as mentioned earlier, the two hormones that help maintain a balanced (homeostatic) blood glucose level are glucagon and insulin. The pancreatic alpha cells produce the glucagon and the beta cells produce the insulin. Too little sugar and we see more glucagon being released, too much and we see more insulin being released. The body's inability to maintain this homeostatic balance happens when the pancreatic beta cells start underperforming or get killed off. Not enough beta cells, means little to no insulin. We can still control too little glucose but the body has no way of controlling too much glucose and this is where major problems start!

Type-1 diabetes

In this particular type of diabetes the exact causes are not known. It is believed to have origins in the genetic disposition of a person, and is usually found rearing its ugly head early on in life. It is most often found before the age of 40 and generally starts in a person's teenage years. Commonly referred to as "Insulin-dependent" diabetes, this is the least common of the two.

How it happens: For unknown reasons, the body's immune system attacks the insulin producing beta cells of the pancreas. Without the beta cells to produce insulin, the body cannot control excessive amounts of glucose in the blood. Modern medical science has produced ways for Type-1 diabetics to help their systems maintain control. The most common method used is self-administered insulin injections.

Once these beta cells in the pancreas have disappeared, the problem becomes permanent and cannot be reversed, it can however been managed.

Type-2 diabetes

The more common of the two, this form starts out in a slightly different way. The same pancreatic beta cells start underperforming. Either too little insulin is produced or as sometimes happens, the body just stops responding to the little insulin that is actually released. It is safe to say that this insulin-resistance is commonly caused by the body having too much sugar for too long, or massive bursts of sugar that the body just cannot handle over a long period of time. This is the connection to the type of food we eat, how we eat, when we eat. Additionally, stress is dealt with using a chemical called cortisol. When we are heavily stressed, cortisol is released which triggers a release of even more glucose. This is how stress is seen as a driver in the list of diabetes causes. Prolonged stress, causes prolonged elevated levels of cortisol, resulting in blood glucose level imbalances.

Type-2 diabetes is commonly dubbed "Insulin-resistant diabetes" because the body has to adapt to the imbalance. There are other forms of this Type-2 based diabetes such as Gestational diabetes that specifically affect pregnant women. The process and results are the same as type-2 diabetes in that the body becomes unable to handle the excessively high levels of glucose in the body. This happens during certain pregnancies and if carefully managed will leave both the mother and child without complications once the pregnancy is over.

Hyperglycemic vs. hypoglycemic

Now this is an aspect of diabetes that can confuse people. Especially when faced with a situation where you need to help a diabetic, it is very important to understand the difference. It could potentially mean life or death. *Hypoglycemia is when there is too little sugar in the blood (low glucose in the blood)Hyperglycemia is when there is too much sugar in the blood (high glucose in the blood)*

<u>Hypoglycemia</u> is usually associated with diabetic's who are on medication. This can be either by taking medication orally or having to administer their insulin. Known as an "insulin reaction" this happens when insulin is at its highest levels in the blood causing the body to reduce blood sugar levels. Sometimes this blood sugar level reduction go's too far and overshoots leaving a diabetic person without enough sugar in their blood. This is a major problem as the human brain uses glucose almost exclusively for fuel. With no glucose available for the brain it begins to starve and you end up with the following symptoms:

Hypoglycemic symptoms:

-Anxiety
-Sweating
-Trembling
-Increased heart rate
-Inability to think clearly
-Headache
-Sleepiness

If not treated hypoglycemia starts with confusion and eventually leads to coma and convulsions. This type of reaction also normally happens very quickly, in as little as a couple of minutes. To treat this rapidly developing emergency it's a simple case of taking in sugar very quickly. A glass of sugar water, a chocolate bar, a couple of sugar cubes. This will allow the body to re-establish homeostasis and for the diabetic person to normalize again.

Hyperglycemia is the essentially the opposite. Being too much sugar (blood glucose level being too high) this affects both Type-1 and Type-2 diabetes patients. The body is unable to control the excessively high level of sugar in the blood and if left untreated this could potentially end with the patient going into coma. Hyperglycemia affects Type-1 & Type-2 patients slightly differently but the end result is the same if not corrected.

Hyperglycemic symptoms:

-Increased thirst
-Needing to urinate constantly
-Dry mouth and skin
-Nausea and vomiting
-Drowsiness and no appetite.

Treatment of Hyperglycemia depends on the type of diabetic you are. It is best to follow the guidance of a professional GP and have a personal care plan as these treatments can vary widely. The best treatment is prevention. Essentially though, for Type-1 diabetics it requires additional insulin intake. For Type-2 diabetics it requires additional physical activity or reduction of sugar (glucose) intake including carbohydrates and increasing the insulin levels in the body.

Chapter 3-what to do

Habit and how to change / reprogram your mind:

The human mind is a complex beast and our behavior even more so. During the course of growing up we develop and learn certain behavior patterns. Such as waking up in the morning, having breakfast, having lunch and then having dinner. These behavior patterns extend to the kinds of things we like to eat and those that we don't. Eating something that you really like on a regular basis is a habit. Smoking is a habit. Brushing your teeth is a habit. These behavior patterns become more deeply ingrained in our minds and lifestyle the more we consistently do them. This makes no difference to whether these are good habits, or bad habits. Logically it follows that habits can be recognized, defined, and changed. The classic example is someone who stops smoking. You could develop a good habit such as exercising regularly if it is not something you've done often before.

Essentially, humans have the ability to program and reprogram their own minds and especially their own behavior patterns. Sometimes we are forced to make these changes, as is the case with a recently diagnosed diabetic. Depending on how you've lived before, there may be some very big changes you need to make. If you are a pre-diabetic and are not quiet there yet, you also need to start making the changes. So how do some people do it so easily and others struggle so much?

Small incremental habitual change:

Generally this is referred to as pure will power. But everyone's life, pressures, strengths and weaknesses are all unique and different. They may be similar but they are all still different. The process can be described as two-fold. You are breaking down and un-learning the habit you wish to stop. It is then best to replace this and learn a new habit that you need or want to have. An example would be cutting out high amounts of sugar in your diet. A persons "sweet tooth" is a natural inclination towards types of sugars, but the regular consumption of those sugars is a habit. This is what can be changed.

If you take your tea and coffee with two sugars, start by dropping it to one sugar for a week and then drop it to none. You will have a couple of weeks where everything tastes terrible but you get used to it and the habit of not eating sugar develops and gets stronger. It is purely a process of repetition and the more you do it the easier it becomes.

To make it easier, list all the things that you need to change and track your progress and how well your doing for at least the first two months, this gives the new behavior patterns / habits time to develop and feel more natural as you keep tight control of them. Ask friends or close family to support you by being involved in the changes your making. The added benefit of including other people in the changes you make is that you now have an intrinsic level of accountability to stay on track.

Immediate change:

Faced with a situation where you have to make immediate changes for the sake of your health can be very hard. No one said it is easy. As with making gradual incremental change, use the same method of tracking and monitoring the changes you are making. Make a list of the changes you need to make. Such as dietary, lifestyle and exercise changes. Learn how to read your body so as to know when you are approaching a limit. Then track and monitor how things are going. Note when you've had difficulties trying not to do something and what caused them.

For example, when you are stressed you may always have something sweet to eat. Try finding an alternative thing to do when you are stressed. Have a couple of glasses of water. Again as mentioned before, involve your friends or family as this gives you the benefit of having those close to you supporting you, and also being accountable makes it easier to stay on track.

Chapter 4-Changes – DIET

What not to eat:

First thing is first. Controlling your blood sugar levels is the "end-game" when having diabetes and controlling your diet. It is about understanding what you are actually eating, and consciously controlling that to make sure you do not overload with food types that will cause your blood sugar levels to spike. The main groups to pay close attention to fall into the following categories: fats, carbohydrates and sodium. Carbohydrates in particular need to be watched, as these are the main source of glucose.

Essentially the body takes carbohydrates and during digestion breaks them down into glucose to be used by the body for fuel. Carbohydrates have been classified in various ways over the years however the most accurate way is by identifying the *glycemic-index* of the carbohydrates you are eating. This is the speed at which carbohydrates can be digested and turned into glucose. In the case of a high glycemic-index, this process happens very quickly and your blood sugar level can spike. This is not ideal! The ideal scenario is when this process happens gradually which equates to eating carbohydrates that digest at a slower rate. There are numerous resources available that will allow you to identify the different food types by their glycemic-index and rate foods on a scale of 1 – 100. The following examples will give you an idea.

High glycemic-index foods: (20+)

-Fried chips / French fries
-Candy bars / refined chocolates
-Rice
-White flour (and the products made using white flour)

Medium glycemic-index foods: (11-19)

-Oats
-Wholegrain breads
-Wholegrain flour (and the products made using wholegrain flour)

Low glycemic-index foods: (Less than 10)

-Beans
-Lentils
-Various nuts (without salt)
-Bran cereals.

Sodium (table salt) is another culprit and it has the following negative effect. An excess of salt causes the body to retain water and subsequently leads to high blood pressure. The connection comes for diabetics, because high blood pressure leads to heart problems and is a common complication of Type-2 diabetes. Too much salt adds to this, compounding the problem and increasing the risk. Too much salt is not a good thing at the best of times, but especially so for a diabetic.

Fats, or more specifically *"saturated fats"* & *"trans fats"* are also widely recognized as having a very strong influence on the risk of cardiovascular problems because they cause high levels of cholesterol. In the same way that sodium can compound the risk of heart complications in Type-2 diabetes, excessive intake of saturated fats will have the same end result, just in a different way. So again, too much saturated fat is not a good idea. Examples of "bad fats" that should be carefully watched are:

Saturated Fats

-Chocolates
-High fat dairy products (full fat cheese / ice cream / sour cream)
-High fat meat / poultry products especially if salted (bacon/processed meats)

Trans Fats

-Margarine
-Processed deep fried foods / French fries
-Heavily processed foods such as crisps / chips / cookies

The idea is to start making sure that you have a balanced diet, but more specifically that your diet does not include high amounts of the products mentioned above, if at all!

Note: This does not mean cut out all fats. This will be explained in the next chapter.

What to replace and what to start eating:

Start with fats, there a certain groups of fats that your body needs and if you cut out all fat, your diet will in fact become unbalanced. So the types of fats you need to keep in your diet in the right amounts are monounsaturated fats, polyunsaturated fats and Omega-3 fatty acids such as:

Monounsaturated fats

-Olive oil / olives
-Nuts / sesame seeds

Polyunsaturated fats

-Nuts
-Vegetable oils
-Soybean

Omega-3 Fatty Acids

-Various types of fish
-Tofu / soybean / flaxseed / canola

Your body needs Carbohydrates, as it is the fuel that your body uses but you need to choose the type of carbohydrates you eat very carefully. The good carbohydrates also contain high amounts of fiber, protein and nutrients, which your body needs. The added benefit of these additional components is that they help to control blood sugar levels by slowing the digestion and absorption of the carbohydrate. As we mentioned before, it is better to have a gradual rise in blood sugar, which your body can respond to and can be controlled.

The healthy Carb choices

-Lentils & Beans
-Whole grain products such as whole-wheat pasta
-Oatmeal
-Sweet potatoes
-Vegetables
-Fresh un-processed fruit

With this brief introduction to what should and should not be a part of a balanced diet specifically for diabetics, this overview should arm you with enough knowledge to start you on the journey to learning about what will be good for you. In particular, seeking out the advice of a professional regarding your own condition is an absolute must. Once you have started along this road, it will eventually become second nature, both in maintaining your own balanced diet and knowing what works for you and what does not. As the 19th century expression goes:

"Give a man a fish and you feed him for a day; Show him how to catch fish and you feed him for a lifetime"

Chapter 5-Your 3-week diabetes countdown program

Step-1

Fear of fat – The change: You need to start thinking about the difference   between good fats and bad fats, cutting out the bad fats entirely but making sure you still get enough of the good fats.

Fear of missing carbs - The change: You need to cut out all the heavy complex carbohydrates especially the ones that have a glycemic index of more than 20. You will still keep some carbohydrates in your diet but this is to balance what you eat and these will be the healthy ones.

Cutting down carbohydrates and increasing the good fats -The change: When cutting down on carbohydrates you will inevitably start feeling hungrier than usual, however this is compensated for by having a slightly higher level of the good fats. Your body will not store these smaller amounts of the good fats, especially if there is no sugar around. This causes the body to start turning to the fats stored in your body and encourages it to start burning these up for fuel instead.

Cutting down on salt and refined sugar - The change: Cutting out salt and refined sugar is a habit you will need to add to the changes in your diet. Cooking without them, not using them on your meals and consciously avoiding foods with high sodium and refined sugar content.

When you eat – The change: Eating regularly and consistently has two main effects. First, your body knows when to expect its next meal and so when you do eat your body is already preparing. If you eat at irregular times and for example have one massive meal a day at different times, your body does not know when the next meal is coming and so go's into a sort of survival mode, storing fat for a rainy day. You do not want your body doing this. Secondly, by increasing the number of meals you have, but decreasing the size and content of your meals you will kick start your metabolism into burning at a higher rate especially with the addition of exercise. This is good because again your body will turn to burning the fat stores you already have instead of storing them. The main upside of this is that you will have steady controllable rises in your blood sugar levels that become manageable by your body instead of the huge sugar spikes.

Step-2

Start by using this template menu to base your new diet on. In the first week you can follow this menu closely, and as the following weeks go by you can start to substitute your own alternatives of the same types into the same categories.

Changing your cooking oil: Use organic cold pressed coconut oil or a healthy alternative to processed vegetable oils to cook with. Only use a dash and stay completely away from any form of deep fried food altogether.

Changing your salad dressing: It is quick and easy to make your own salad dressing with extra virgin olive oil, fresh lemon juice and a dash of salt. You can also make a small balsamic dressing. Do not use dressings, which you buy in the shop, as their refined sugar contents are excessively high.

Steam vegetables: Boiling vegetables will strip them of all their goodness and flavor. Steaming for a short time so they are hot but not soft and soggy, keeps all their goodness and keeps their texture and flavor as well.

Salads: Be inventive. Use vegetables, use fruit, use nuts in small amounts and you can even spice them up with very small amounts of a good strong cheese. An especially good way to make food and in particular salads, is to use color! Red peppers, tomatoes, yellow peppers, fresh beetroot etc. We eat with our eyes as well as our mouths!

Drinks: Avoid soda's, soft drinks, processed drinks, fruit juices etc. They have excessively high levels of sugar. This includes your standard coffee from the big coffee shop brands! A flavored latte from one of the big brands with all the trimmings can contain as much sugar as eating a candy bar, slice of cake and a soft drink combined.

Water: The importance of water can never be over emphasized and it is especially important to maintaining a healthy diet. An easy tip is to drink a glass of water every time you have a hunger pang in between meals, every time you want to eat something sweet and every time you want to have something that you now know is not healthy for your diet. Build the habit of having a glass of water as your new preference.

WEEK 1

Monday:

Breakfast: Omelet: mixed vegetables cooked in butter or coconut oil.

Lunch: Cup of natural unflavored Yogurt with blueberries and a handful of almonds (unsalted).

Dinner: Beef burger with cheese (no bun), mixed steamed vegetables.

Tuesday:

Breakfast: 2 x Bacon strips and 2 x boiled eggs.

Lunch: White chicken breast cooked with steamed mixed vegetables.

Dinner: Salmon fillet with olive oil and mixed steamed vegetables.

Wednesday:

Breakfast: 2 x boiled eggs with olive oil, small salad and fresh olives.

Lunch: Seafood salad with olive oil. (do not use processed salad dressings!!).

Dinner: 2 x grilled chicken fillets with mixed steamed vegetables.

Thursday:

Breakfast: Tuna omelet with various vegetables cooked in olive oil or coconut oil.

Lunch: 1 x cup vegetable soup.

Dinner: 250g lean steak and mixed steamed vegetables.

Friday:

Breakfast: 2 x bacon strips and 2 x boiled eggs.

Lunch: White chicken breast salad with some olive oil.

Dinner: Steamed fresh fish fillets with mixed steamed vegetables.

Saturday:

Breakfast: Omelet: mixed vegetables cooked in butter or coconut oil.

Lunch: Natural unflavored yogurt with berries, coconut flakes and a handful of walnuts.

Dinner: Grilled chicken breast with fresh spinach, onion and walnut salad.

Sunday:

Breakfast: 2 x bacon strips and 2 x boiled Eggs.

Lunch: Smoothie with milk, flavored protein powder and mixed fresh berries.

Dinner: Minute steak with mixed steamed vegetables.

WEEK 2

Monday:

Breakfast: Omelet: with chopped bacon in olive oil or coconut oil.

Lunch: White chicken breast salad with some olive oil.

Dinner: 2 grilled fresh fish fillets with mixed steamed vegetables.

Tuesday:

Breakfast: 2 x bacon strips and 2 x boiled eggs.

Lunch: Grilled white chicken breast salad with olive oil.

Dinner: Salmon fillet with olive oil and mixed steamed vegetables.

Wednesday:

Breakfast: 2 x boiled eggs with extra virgin olive oil, small salad and fresh olives.

Lunch: Seafood salad with extra virgin olive oil. (Do not use processed salad dressings!!).

Dinner: 2 x grilled chicken fillets with steamed vegetables.

Thursday:

Breakfast: Tuna omelet: fresh tomatoes cooked in butter or coconut oil.

Lunch: 1 x cup vegetable soup.

Dinner: 250g lean steak and mixed steamed vegetables.

Friday:

Breakfast: 2 x bacon strips and 2 x boiled eggs.

Lunch: White chicken breast salad with some extra virgin olive oil.

Dinner: Steamed fresh fish fillets with mixed steamed vegetables.

Saturday:

Breakfast: Omelet: mixed vegetables cooked in olive oil or coconut oil.

Lunch: Natural unflavored yogurt with berries, mixed (unsalted) nuts.

Dinner: Grilled chicken breast with fresh spinach, onion and walnut salad.

Sunday:

> **Breakfast:** 2 x bacon strips and 2 x boiled eggs.

> **Lunch:** Smoothie with milk, flavored protein powder and mixed fresh berries.
> **Dinner:** Minute steak with mixed

steamed   vegetables.

WEEK 3

Monday:

> **Breakfast:** 1 x cup of oats, milk and dash of honey.

> **Lunch:** Tuna salad with fresh mixed salad leaves and olive oil.

> **Dinner:** Grilled minute steak with steamed mixed vegetables.

Tuesday:

> **Breakfast:** 2 x boiled eggs with extra

virgin olive oil and fresh tomato salad.

Lunch: Grilled white chicken breast salad with olive oil.

Dinner: Salmon fillet with olive oil and mixed steamed vegetables.

Wednesday:

Breakfast: 2 x boiled eggs with olive oil, small salad and fresh olives.

Lunch: Seafood salad with olive oil. (Do not use processed salad dressings!!).

Dinner: 2 x grilled chicken fillets with steamed vegetables.

Thursday:

Breakfast: Omelet with mixed vegetables cooked in butter or coconut oil.
Lunch: 1 x cup vegetable soup.

Dinner: 1 x beef cheese burger (no bread / fries) and mixed steamed vegetables.

Friday:

Breakfast: 2 x bacon strips and 2 x boiled eggs.

Lunch: White chicken breast salad with some olive oil.

Dinner: Grilled fresh fish fillets with mixed steamed vegetables.

Saturday:

Breakfast: Omelet: mixed vegetables cooked in butter or coconut oil.

Lunch: Natural unflavored yogurt with fresh mixed fruit.

Dinner: Grilled chicken breast with fresh spinach, onion and walnut salad.

Sunday:

Breakfast: Muesli, fresh unflavored yoghurt, fresh fruit and dash of honey.

Lunch: Smoothie with milk, flavored

DAY	Breakfast	Snack	Lunch	Snack	Dinner
Monday	YES	Nuts and fruit	YES	Cup of coffee	YES
Tuesday	-	-	-	-	-
Wednesday	-	-	-	-	-
Thursday	-	-	-	-	-
Friday	-	-	-	-	-
Saturday	-	-	-	-	-
Sunday	-	-	-	-	-

protein powder and mixed fresh berries.

Dinner: Minute steak with mixed steamed vegetables.

Keep a diary: The purpose of keeping a daily diary for at least the first three weeks is to help you stay on top of the new diet plan if you are having a hard time sticking to it. This is also a way for you to see where you have had the most difficulty and best successes. You will also be able to see what you have achieved on a daily basis. And as you start clocking up more days successfully completed, your confidence and resolve strengthens and grows.

Keeping a simple daily diary of what you've been eating is as much psychological as it is a planning tool.

When using this table for all three weeks, for breakfast, lunch and dinner just make a note if you have had the meal from the meal plan or not. If not then make sure you make a note of the extra things you've had or the alternatives that you've substituted in. For the snack sections use this to keep an eye on those extra little things you have during the course of the day. It is the chocolate bars, biscuits, processed snacks, and drinks that can also make a big impact on your sugar levels.

Chapter 6-25 delicious super-food recipes to help you

5 breakfast Super food Recipes:

1) ***Breakfast Omelet***

Whisk up two eggs with mixed herbs and then pour into a pan that has a dash of cold pressed coconut oil in it. Then add ½ cup of chopped fresh mushrooms and chopped red peppers. To create a fluffy omelet you can add a dash of milk when you are whisking it up. Serve with fresh flat leaf parsley and a few slices of fresh tomato.

-2 x eggs
-mixed herbs
-1/4 teaspoon cold pressed organic coconut oil, / extra virgin olive oil
-1/4 cup fresh chopped mushrooms
-1/2 fresh chopped pepper (red / yellow / green peppers)

2) ***Muesli breakfast*** –

Layer a ¼ cup of Muesli (natural muesli without all the extra trimmings), fresh berries especially blueberries (diabetic super food) and fresh natural Greek yoghurt (unflavored). If you absolutely need to you can add a dash of honey but try and avoid sweet sugars during the first 3 weeks especially.

-1/4 cup natural muesli (without extra trimmings such as berries and chocolate and flavorings)
-1/3 cup mixed fresh berries (blueberries if you can get them)
-1/4 cup natural Greek yoghurt (unflavored and no added fruits or trimmings)

3) ***Scrambled eggs***

Whisk 2 eggs up with mixed herbs and a dash of milk. Pour into a pan which is pre-heated with a dash of cold pressed coconut oil / extra virgin olive oil. Cook and scramble the eggs until done to your liking. Finely chop 1 fresh tomato with a ¼ fresh onion and mix up into a small salad. For a dressing use a dash of olive oil, fresh lemon juice and a pinch of salt to flavor.

-2 x eggs

-mixed herbs
-1/4 teaspoon cold pressed organic coconut oil, / extra virgin olive oil
-dash of milk
-1 fresh tomato chopped
-1/4 fresh onion chopped
-home made dressing (dash olive oil / dash fresh lemon juice / pinch of salt)

4) ***Oats bowl***

½ cup of organic rolled oats with a ½ cup boiled water. Microwave for 2 minutes then stir. Microwave again for another two minutes and serve with ¼ cup almond / soymilk and a ¼ cup fresh berries.

-1/2cup rolled organic oats
-1/2 cup fresh water
-1/4 cup almond / soymilk
-1/4 cup fresh berries

5) ***Smoothie***

Take a ¼ cup fresh natural Greek yoghurt, handful fresh berries and table spoon of organic peanut butter and blend together. You can increase the size of the smoothie by adding ¼ cup of water without increasing additional fat / calorie amounts.

-1/4 cup fresh Greek yoghurt
-1/2 cup fresh berries
-table spoon peanut butter / handful of unsalted nuts
-1/4 cup water

5 Lunch super food recipes:

1) ***Tuna Salad***

fresh lettuce / spinach / romaine lettuce as the base, add chopped tomato, chopped onion, chopped yellow peppers and chopped celery. Then add drained tuna in spring water (don't use the tuna in brine because of the additional salt). Make a fresh homemade dressing with extra virgin olive oil, balsamic, mixed herbs and fresh lemon juice.

-can tuna in spring water
-mix green salad leaves

-1 fresh tomato
-1/4 chopped onion
-1/2 chopped yellow pepper
-2 sticks fresh chopped celery
-dash extra virgin olive oil, balsamic, fresh lemon juice and a pinch of salt

2) *Lunch wrap*

Use a whole grain wrap and fill it with sliced roast beef, fresh tomato, flat leaf parsley, fresh chopped tomato, sundried tomato, sprinkle of chopped chill peppers, mixed herbs and a dash of feta cheese.

-1 x medium whole grain wrap
-1/2 fresh sliced tomato
-handful fresh chopped flat leaf parsley
-couple of chopped sundried tomatoes
-1 or 2 small fresh chopped chili peppers, this is to personal preference
-sprinkle of mixed herbs
-dash of crumbled feta cheese to add extra flavor

3) *Salad meal*

Using cooked quinoa as the base, you can add, sundried tomatoes, fresh chopped parsley, sliced carrots, and cut up steamed broccoli / green beans. To top this off you can add a fresh homemade dressing of extra virgin olive oil, lemon juice, pinch of salt and mixed herbs.

-1/2 cup cooked quinoa
-handful chopped sundried tomatoes
-fresh chopped parsley, sliced carrots
-cup of steamed broccoli and green beans
-home made dressing of extra virgin olive oil, fresh lemon juice, pinch of salt and pinch of mixed herbs

4) *Grilled chicken salad*

1 breast of grilled chicken, in a salad of mixed lettuce, cucumber, celery, fresh mint, onion, spring onion, chopped red and yellow pepper topped with a homemade fresh dressing and a sprinkle of parmesan cheese.

-1 grilled, sliced chicken breast
-fresh mixed salad leaves (romaine, iceberg and Boston bib lettuce / young spinach)
-1/2 cup chopped spring onion, cucumber and celery
-handful of fresh chopped mint
-1/4 cup fresh chopped peppers (mixed)
-sprinkle of parmesan cheese shavings
-home made dressing of extra virgin olive oil, balsamic, mixed herbs and dash of salt

5) *Roast beef couscous salad*

using steamed organic couscous add lean cooked diced roast beef, chopped red / yellow peppers, sprinkle of chili flakes and finely chopped fresh tomato. Use a homemade dressing of olive oil, fresh lemon juice and a dash of salt and pepper. You can also add a sprinkle of dried berries to create a contrasting flavor.

-left over roast beef chopped up
-cup of cooked organic couscous
-1/2 chopped red and yellow pepper
-mixed herbs and dried chili flakes
-1 finely chopped fresh tomato

-extra virgin olive oil, dash fresh lemon juice, pinch of salt

-small helping of raisin / dried berries

10 Dinner super food recipes:

3)   *Tuna steak grilled*

1 tuna steak (250g) grilled with a light drizzle of extra virgin olive oil and mixed herbs. Served with steamed mixed vegetables such as fresh green asparagus and spinach lightly tossed with onion and garlic in the pan. The asparagus should be blanched / steamed slightly so as to rctain their crunchiness, goodness and flavor. The spinach leaves can be tossed and sautéed lightly in a pan with a dash of olive oil, fresh chopped onion and   fresh chopped garlic.

-1 x 250g tuna steak

-dash of olive oil for the steak and for the tossed sautéed spinach

-handful of fresh green asparagus, very lightly steamed

-small bag of spinach leaves-1 garlic clove

-1/2 fresh onion

-mixed herbs to add flavor

2) *Salmon fillets with Indian spice*

2 small salmon fillets rubbed with Indian spices (including turmeric) lightly baked. Serve this with a ½ cup of cooked quinoa mixed with finely chopped sundried tomatoes and mixed herbs. You can also add a small salad of fresh chopped tomato and onion, served with fresh flat leaf parsley, mint and a home made dressing of olive oil, fresh lemon juice and a dash of salt and mixed herbs

-250g of salmon fillet rubbed with Indian spice

-1/2 cup cooked quinoa
-handful of sundried tomatoes
-mixed herbs
-1 fresh chopped tomato
-1/2 fresh chopped onion
-handful fresh flat leaf parsley and mint

3) *Calamari and fish fillets in lemon and Cajun spice*

Baby Patagonian calamari with diced chunks of fresh fish fillets, lightly tossed in the pan with cold pressed organic coconut oil, fresh lemon juice and Cajun spices. Serve this with a mixed salad of blanched mixed vegetables (asparagus / green beans), lettuce, onion, fresh basil leaves, and a light citrus dressing of lemon, orange juice and extra virgin olive oil.

-150g fresh Patagonian calamari
-150g of diced sea bass / bream (you can use a local fish of your choice)
-1/2 teaspoon of organic cold pressed coconut oil
-Cajun spices including chili
-handful of green beans and fresh green asparagus
-handful of fresh chopped lettuce and fresh basil leaves
-1/2 fresh chopped onion
-dash of fresh lemon juice and fresh orange juice
-dash of extra virgin olive oil
-mixed herbs to taste

4)   *Steamed monkfish & cherry tomatoes*

Monkfish tale, baked with garlic, mixed herbs and cherry tomatoes. Serve this with sliced grilled eggplant. You can also serve a small spinach leaf salad with fresh chopped onion and walnuts dressed with a light citrus dressing.

-250g monkfish tail
-sliced, grilled eggplant
-1 fresh chopped garlic clove
-handful fresh cherry tomatoes
-small bag fresh spinach leaves
-1/2 fresh chopped onion
-handful fresh walnuts (unsalted)
-dash of extra virgin olive oil
-dash of fresh lemon and orange juice
-mixed herbs

5)   *Steamed bream (foil bag)*

Whole bream, steamed in a foil bag/envelope with garlic, mixed mushrooms, cherry tomatoes, basil and mixed herbs. When served you can have this with a light green leaf salad topped with an olive oil and fresh lemon juice dressing.

-whole bream fish
-1 chopped garlic clove
-assorted mixed exotic mushroom (chestnut, shitake mushrooms)
-fresh cherry tomatoes
-basil and mixed herbs
-tablespoon of olive oil for steaming the fish
-extra virgin olive oil and fresh lemon juice with a pinch of salt for the salad dressing
-mixed green salad leaves

6) ***Roast beef***

silverside / topside / rump roast. Roast in the oven with fresh black mushrooms topped with herbs and a small helping of feta cheese on the mushrooms. You can serve this with steamed mixed vegetables (broccoli, cauliflower, asparagus).

-roast (as big as you like as you can use the leftover cold meat for lunch and snacks during the rest of the week)
-large black mushrooms

-mixed herbs for the roast and the black mushroom topping
-1/4 cup feta cheese for the mushroom topping
-handful of broccoli and a handful of cauliflower steamed

7) ***Minute steak***

2 minute steaks lightly seared in the pan with a ¼ teaspoon organic pressed coconut oil and cracked black pepper. Serve this with either a light mixed salad or a portion of fresh sautéed spinach, onion and garlic. Dress the salad with a homemade dressing of extra virgin olive oil, fresh lemon juice and a pinch of salt.

-250g minute steak (lean)
-1/4 teaspoon of organic cold pressed coconut oil to sear the steaks with
-small packet of fresh baby spinach leaves
-1/2 chopped garlic clove
-1 fresh chopped onion
-mixed herbs and cracked black pepper
-extra virgin olive oil
-fresh lemon juice for the dressing
-mixed fresh salad leaves for the salad

8) *Grilled chicken breast*

Grilled white chicken breast covered in mixed herbs and Cajun spice. Serve with cooked quinoa, fresh chopped chives and mixed herbs. Include a small fresh spinach leaf salad with a dash of olive oil and balsamic.

-2 chicken breast (white – no skin)
-mixed herbs and Cajun spice
-1/2 cup cooked quinoa
-fresh chopped chives
-handful of fresh baby spinach leaves
-extra virgin olive oil and dash of balsamic vinegar

9) *Chicken curry (Thai)*

diced white chicken breast simmered in a sauce of fresh yoghurt, coconut milk and mixed Thai spices. Include galangal as one of the spice ingredients to give a slight lemon finish. Fresh chopped vegetables such as carrot, sugar snap peas, bamboo shoots, yellow peppers and baby white mushrooms. You can have this as   is or you can have a small serving of organic brown rice with it.

-2 diced white chicken breasts
-1 small pot fresh unflavored yoghurt
-1/2 tin of organic coconut milk
-mixed Thai spices (including ginger and galangal)
-mixed chopped fresh vegetables (carrots / bamboo shoots / sugar snap peas / yellow peppers)
-cup of baby white mushrooms
-1/2 cup of organic brown rice

10) ***Stir-fry (chicken / beef)***

diced white chicken or lean beef lightly stir-fried with fresh chopped mixed vegetables and a 1/2 teaspoon of organic cold pressed coconut milk. This is a very quick meal to prepare and remember not to overcook the vegetables. They should just be heated and must remain crunchy. It is not necessary to serve this with a starch so feel free to have a nice large helping if you do not have a starch with it.

-2 white chicken breast diced / 200g lean beef diced

-fresh chopped mixed vegetables (red & yellow peppers / carrots / sugar snap peas / spring onion / bamboo shoots / Bok-Choi)
-1/2 teaspoon of organic cold pressed coconut oil
-mixed herbs

Snacks

Snacks are what tend to catch a lot of people because the kinds of things that are usually chosen end up having very high amounts of sugar. Ideally try and stick to fresh / unprocessed foods if you are going to snack and consciously make sure that you only have two very small snacks a day, in between your main meals.

5 snack options:

1) ***Nuts***

Mixed nuts are a very good source of protein and essential oils. However use them with caution and only have a small handful at the most every other day. Do not use the processed / roasted / salted kinds. Plain is the best way to go.

2) **_Yoghurt_**

In small amounts yoghurt is particular good for two reasons. It contains bio-cultures that help keep your stomach healthy and working properly. It also contains casein that is a very slow release source of energy. However be very careful of flavored yoghurts, as they will contain high amounts of sugars and artificial food products.

3) **_Beef Jerky / Biltong_**

Cured dried meat depending on the type that you buy will be a great lean source of protein and will help fill in the gap between your main meals.

4) **_Protein shakes_**

This is not meant as a meal replacement but as a small snack. Especially if you are starting a regimen of exercise, getting that extra boost of protein for your body will prevent your body catabolizing your muscle when you shift onto a low calorie diet.

5) *__Water__*

This may sound like a very odd thing to suggest, but when you have those hunger pangs or urges in between main meals, a large glass of water or three will do wonders. It fills you up, your body can never have enough water and the host of benefits in keeping your body hydrated, flushed and detoxed are just a few of the wonderful effects good old water has for our bodies.

Chapter 7-conclusion

Now that you have been given an overview, it is time to conclude this guide to reversing diabetes by finalizing the key points. If you are a Type-2 diabetic it is possible to reverse your diabetes. This can be done by taking yourself onto a strict diet for a minimum of three weeks to start the process of normalizing bodily imbalances. In extreme cases restricting your diet to below your average daily requirement, strictly sticking to protein, vegetables and a small amount of healthy fats speeds this process up. Then you will start to understand what your body needs. From this point you can then modify your diet to give your body what it needs to stay healthy and not just what you feel like eating. By taking your body off sugar and high amounts of unhealthy carbohydrates you will reduce the effect these high levels of blood sugar and blood sugar spikes are having. This gives your body a chance to normalize itself.

The main goal for your body is twofold. Firstly, to drastically reduce the levels of sugar in your body. Secondly to kick start your metabolism into burning fat instead of storing it. You want to burn off all that excess fat, especially as your body will start to burn the fat around your organs first. Ideally we want the fat removed from being anywhere near your pancreas. You will develop habits that control your new healthy balanced diet. With changing your lifestyle habits you will start to benefit from being stronger, fitter and healthier through the increased physical activity you undertake. On top of all of these new benefits you will start enjoying, your body will start to normalize and the "condition" of being diabetic will disappear. Good luck and stick with it, you will thank yourself for years to come.